STEM CELL
BANKING

ALL YOU SHOULD KNOW ABOUT

MITCH SHAH

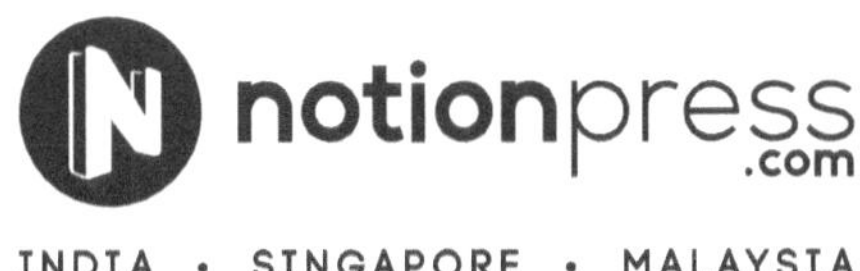

INDIA • SINGAPORE • MALAYSIA

Notion Press

Old No. 38, New No. 6
McNichols Road, Chetpet
Chennai – 600 031

First Published by Notion Press 2019
Copyright © Mitch Shah 2019
All Rights Reserved.

ISBN 978-1-64650-561-6

This book has been published with all efforts taken to make the material error–free after the consent of the author. However, the author and the publisher do not assume and hereby disclaim any liability to any party for any loss, damage, or disruption caused by errors or omissions, whether such errors or omissions result from negligence, accident, or any other cause.

While every effort has been made to avoid any mistake or omission, this publication is being sold on the condition and understanding that neither the author nor the publishers or printers would be liable in any manner to any person by reason of any mistake or omission in this publication or for any action taken or omitted to be taken or advice rendered or accepted on the basis of this work. For any defect in printing or binding the publishers will be liable only to replace the defective copy by another copy of this work then available.

Bio

Mitch Shah has a degree in BS, MBA from California, U.S.A. He has worked for companies like NASA and Sony Pictures. He is an entrepreneur, holding offices in several countries, and is a member of many prestigious organizations. He is an avid movie lover, traveler and also keeps himself updated on the latest technological and medical discoveries/inventions. He is a philanthropist and does his best to help society.

For any queries, you can contact him on Instagram @mitchshah

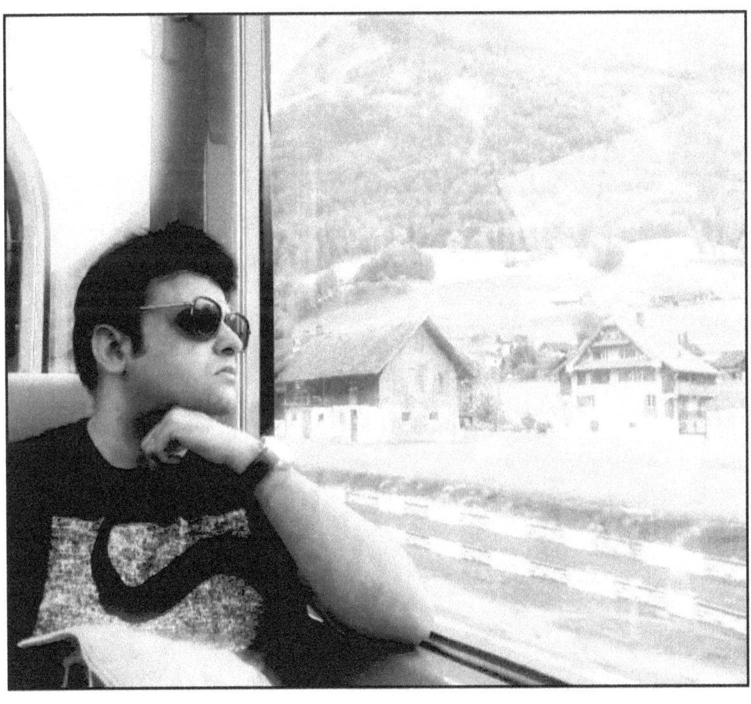

Dedication

I would like to dedicate this book to my dear daughter Jiana, for who this entire journey took place.

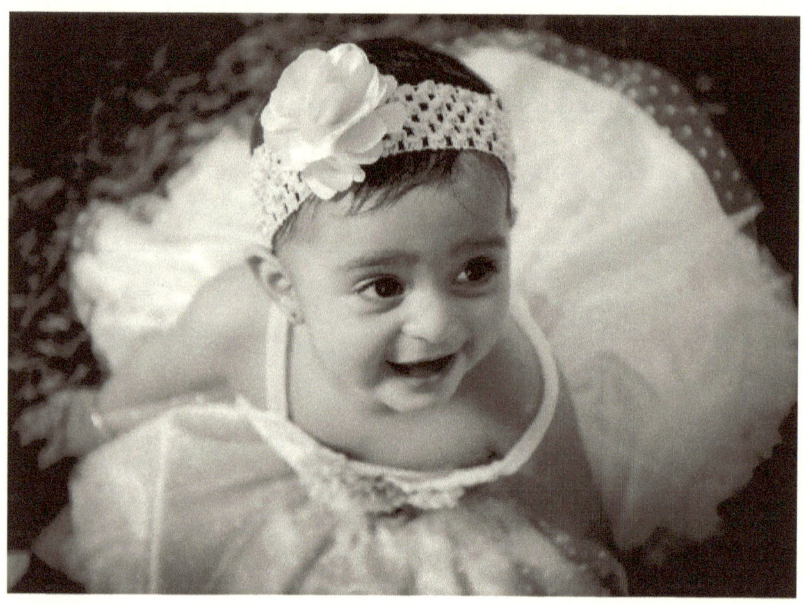

Disclaimer

The book is purely based on the personal experience of the author and is served to help others to avoid hardships that are being faced for Stem Cell Banking. The information given in this book is intended solely for advisory and knowledge purposes and may not be used as a substitute for professional advice and information, as circumstances will vary from person to person. It would be best if you did not act or rely upon this information without seeking professional advice. Do not attempt any of the suggested actions, solutions, remedies, or instructions found in this book without first consulting with a qualified professional. The materials are not intended to be, nor do they constitute actionable professional advice. Transmission of this information is not intended to create a professional-client relationship between the author and you. The author, editors, publisher and other staff associated with this book are not qualified professionals, and are simply aggregating information found online and offline for general knowledge and suggestions. Due credits and references have been given to the sources of the contents of this book. The author apologies for any unintentional typographical and informational errors or omissions in this book.

Contents

Introduction

I was excited, as I was going to be a father. Like any responsible parent, I wanted the absolute best for my baby. I had heard about Stem cell banking and how it's going to be a thing of the future. At first, I asked our Gynaecologist about the best stem cell bank. I was flabbergasted when she told me, "all are good; you can choose any." Next, I asked our family doctor. He thought that Stem cell banking was a scheme to loot people's money. There was no significant use, except a few rare diseases. I was even more shocked and confused. Then I turned towards my friends, who claimed to have done stem cell banking. What followed next was horrifying. All of them went to almost the same companies, which is ok if that was the best company. However, their selection criteria were based on two things:

A) Everyone is going with that company, so it must be good

B) They were earning a Referral bonus, where the first party gets cash and the second party gets a referral discount.

Wow, I could not believe what I was hearing. I mean I go through more research for buying my car than this. I was not going to settle on these ridiculous reasons to decide upon a company that I want to bank my baby/s stem cell with.

So I began to research extensively on the subject both online and offline until I was convinced of my choice of stem cell banking. What I found was: There is so much more to stem cell banking than people realize, especially when your child's future is on stake. Thousands of parents have just given away their money without realizing its long term effects, costs, hidden terms, and conditions. So I decided to share my knowledge by writing this book on All. You should know about Stem Cell Banking.

I. Why Stem Cell Banking?

Science has given us another revolution with the discovery of Stem Cells and the ways that these Stem Cells can change our present and future. Today, there are so many proven cases that we can witness about the success of using our own or matched stem cells for therapies of certain diseases.

Moreover, that's not all; the revolution has just begun.

We are still on our way to finding more about Stem Cells, their use in therapies, and more. Hence, banking the stem cells is like getting a sure-shot Insurance Plan for the entire family, all at once, that will never fail or go for waste.

II. Why Cord Blood Banking?

Following the birth of a baby, the placenta and umbilical cord are usually thrown away along with these life-saving stem cells that can treat many different cancers, immune deficiencies, and genetic disorders.

The umbilical cord is the source of life between the mother and the baby since the fertilization stage until the baby is born. Cord blood is the blood that remains in the placenta and umbilical cord after a baby is born. Cord Blood Cells are stem cells extracted from the umbilical cord blood and placenta after the baby is born and the umbilical cord is cut. The process of collection is without any pain or harm to both the mother and the child as the blood is collected after the umbilical cord is cut, before discarding it as a biological waste product.

The stem cells found in cord blood restore the function of the patient's immune and blood producing systems. It is an alternative to using bone marrow, with the advantage of being immediately available when required.

Cord blood is rich in stem cells and can be used to treat patients who are suffering from life-threatening diseases, including:

- ☐ Malignancies – In Haematological malignancies: Allogeneic stem cell transplant is preferred. This is because there is a definite graft versus Leukemia effect, which gives a therapeutic benefit. This happens only in allogeneic transplants.

- ☐ Bone marrow failure – when the bone marrow doesn't produce the cells it should.

- ☐ Haemoglobinopathies – a blood disorder, e.g. Sickle cell anemia, Thalassaemia

☐ Cannot be cured by own cord blood as it's a genetic condition. **Patients stem cell will have the same genetic problem. However, a disease-free sibling can be the donor**.

☐ Immunodeficiencies – when the immune system doesn't work properly.

☐ Metabolic disorders – which affect the breakdown of waste products in the body.

Thanks to scientific research in this field, we are constantly discovering more and more diseases and conditions that can be successfully treated with stem cells found in cord blood.

*** Kindly refer to the list of curable diseases for further details ***

Important: Today, stem cell Banking is one of the most pathbreaking healthcare insurance decision one can take for self and family. However, the awareness of this particular importance has still not been created. The advantage is very much relative, and statistics are not available, but this field has **tremendous scope for development**.

III. Public Banking Vs. Private Banking

Cord blood Banking can be a priceless investment, and it is very important to choose the right mode of banking the precious stem cells as this is once in a lifetime opportunity, and you do not want to regret later on.

After birth, your baby no longer needs the umbilical cord or placenta, but the blood that remains could be a lifesaver for a patient who needs it, including a member of your own family. That's because this blood is rich with blood-forming stem cells.

Choosing the right Stem Cell Banking service would mean a lot of ground and research work to identify the best possible combination of services and facilities that you want available in the future.

There are two types of Stem Cell Banking available:

a) **Public Banking**: Public Banking would mean donating the stem cells extracted from the umbilical cord blood and umbilical cord tissue of the new-born baby for any **future use for anyone who needs them**. Public Banking **does not involve any cost** to the donor; it is free. Since the stem cells have been donated, the donor loses the right to reserve or claim these stem cells for self and family or even for the child whose stem cells have been donated, in case of any future requirement. Publically Banked Stem Cells are available for either research purpose or therapy/transplants as and when needed (on payment for the same) at the discretion of the governing body which maintains the viability while storing and preserving these stem cells.

In Public Banking, since the secured Stem Cells are not the property of any individual, there are no such particular norms that need to be understood or kept in mind. The donation of stem cells will be done through the hospital directly, where the delivery of the child is taking place if that particular hospital facilitates the same.

The first Public Bank was established in New York in 1993 Cord blood units in public banks can be made available for the patients worldwide. Anyone from any part of the world can access this reserve in a public bank. The registries present worldwide help search for HLA matched specimen. There are no charges for the storage process. However, the recipients who will use the cord blood units for their treatment pay a charge. The list of Public cord blood Bank is in Annexure 1.

b) **Private Banking**: In Private Banking, the Umbilical Cord Blood and Cord Tissues are stored for private use at the time of future needs, if any, reassuring all the rights of ownership. Private Banking has been made more convenient and affordable through different plans and flexible options for payment that are available today. The preserved stem cells can be made available for therapy and transplants for the child, and technically for the child's parents, grandparents or any other family member, friends, or anyone else in need, if the agreement holder decides to donate or use these stem cells in either of the above cases.

When it's a Private bank, the story is different. The cord blood is stored by a family against a specific price. This cord blood can be used by the family if and when needed.

The chances of it ever being used is rare.

1:1000 to 1:200000 (1)

Another point of worry is the quality of cord blood stored in private banks. Are they stored in conditions optimal for future use? Very few people storing cord blood would wish to use them until needed. So the truth of storage quality needs assessment by people not having a conflict of interest.

Facts and myths of private cord blood banking

There is a lot of emotional marketing of private cord blood banking to young and expecting parents. This vulnerable segment feels a sense of responsibility towards their unborn child, and this gets exploited. Even though stem cell transplant is promised as a miracle cure for all ills, there are few truths you must know

1) **Autologous cord stem cell** or one's stem cell cannot be used to cure their own genetic diseases. This includes hemoglobinopathies, storage disorder, and others. The genetic mutation causing the disease in the patient is also present in the patient's stored cord cell.

2) **In Haematologicalmalignancies**: Allogeneic stem cell transplant is preferred. This is because there is a definite graft versus Leukemia effect, which gives a therapeutic benefit. This happens only in allogeneic transplants.

3) **In High-risk solid tumors**, the patients own stored stem cell, or Autologous stem transplant is used. However, **in most cases, stem cells can be harvested from the peripheral blood or bone marrow of the patient**. This will hopefully provide comparable results to that using Umbilical cord blood in several diseases in the near future with further research.

When is a Private bank recommended?

When there is an existing family member (parents or sibling) having a disease approved to be cured by allogeneic stem cell transplant. Like Leukaemia, haemoglobinopathy, bone marrow failure, etc. Thalassemia is a common non-malignant indication for this treatment in India. Important to understand a few points

a) Unaffected sibling needs to be the donor.

b) HLA matching is mandatory

c) **The patients own cord blood or allogeneic stem cell transplant is not possible in Thalassemia.**

d) If stem cell from HLA matched sibling is not stored due to any reason, its still possible to perform a stem cell transplant using peripheral blood stem cells or bone marrow.

e) A single unit of umbilical cord blood cell may be insufficient in an adult.

f) The chance of a unit of cord blood being used in a public bank is higher than in a private bank.

g) The **information spread by private cord blood banks is misleading**. Real case reports and success stories need to be available in a transparent manner before their claims can be given weight. **In countries like France and Italy, any advertisement about Private cord blood banking is illegal**.

For private Banking, there are certain parameters that the preserver's family must seek to understand and confirm before banking the stem cells of their child with a Stem Cell Bank.

In one of our next section, we have listed down a checklist of key points as to what facilities and benefits must be available in a particular Stem Cell Bank, as a referral for the parents-to-be.

*** **Kindly refer to the Points that need to be considered for choosing the Stem Cell Bank** ***

IV. How to Choose the Right Private Stem Cell Bank

Finding a reliable cord blood bank is crucial. If a Cord Blood Bank does not have high standards for handling, shipping, and storing cord blood, your baby's cord blood might not be usable if you ever need it. Moreover, if a bank isn't financially stable, where and how your baby's cord blood is stored long term could be affected.

Cord blood storage is a medical service. So if you shop for a provider based solely on price, for example, the bank you select may not meet the highest quality standards.

While all cord blood banks must pass FDA inspection, beyond that baseline, they vary in their practices and standards. Both the doctors at transplant centres and those conducting clinical trials require cord blood to be tested against rigorous guidelines before it's used for medical therapy. If the day comes when one of your children needs the cord blood, you'll want to feel confident that it was stored properly.

Most Important points to be considered while choosing the Stem Cell Banking Company:

a. How do I begin my search for a good Cord Blood Bank?

Start your research for a goof cord blood bank early. Most cord blood banks urge expectant parents to enroll in their program during the second trimester. Some banks even offer discounts if you sign up early.

(Even in your third trimester, you can still plan to bank your baby's cord blood. But if you're getting close to your due date, you may have to pay a late enrollment fee.)

Here are some tips for getting started:

- ✓ Have a suitable amount of time in hand to visit and review the available services and weigh your options.

- ✓ You need to ensure that your obstetrician and the hospital knows of your decision and knows how to collect cord blood. Many stem cell bank may offer to send their personnel. So check that, as collection time and method is crucial for the viability of the cord blood cells.

- ✓ Review the Find a Family Bank search tool, compiled by the non-profit Parent's Guide to Cord Blood Foundation. Their database contains approximately 200 family cord blood banks worldwide with contact information, descriptions, and price comparison tables and all the other required details for all countries.

- ✓ You can ask friends and family, as well as your healthcare provider, for recommendations. Some family cord blood banks offer financial incentives to customers who refer new parents. However, choose the one you feel most confident about after diligent research.

- ✓ When considering a bank, please don't assume it's best to enroll in one close to your home. The bank's headquarters and its storage facility may be in different locations. What's important is the storage and availability of their services.

b. Decide whether it is worth spending and preserving the stem cells in a private bank instead of a public bank. Is it a NECESSITY or an OPPORTUNITY?

If there is a specific disease that one of your family members is suffering from, and the treatment suggests that a stem cell therapy or transplant is necessary for the same, then **Stem Cell Banking at a private bank** becomes **not just a necessity, but essential.**

In other cases, if the family has a history of distant relatives suffering from an incurable disease, and you expect that the same might or might not occur for your family, stem cell banking can be beneficial in case of such a need.

Alternatively, without any specific disease within the immediate family or an expected family history disease, people can still count on stem cell banking as possible **biological insurance** in some cases. Nothing in this world is predictable, and trouble does not knock before entering your door. With the current ratio of new diseases striking the population and no sign of guaranteed treatments, stem cells are a big hope.

c. Contact all the possible stem cell banks and request for a presentation at your home or any place of your convenience, in front of all the decision making family members.

Collect all possible information from the cord blood bank executives; it would help in comparing and choosing the right stem cell bank as per your understanding.

IMPORTANT: Local stem cell banks are as good as international banks as long as they **have excellent accreditation, transport and storage facilities**, financial banking etc.

d. Check for Accreditation

These are the accreditation standards that your bank must have:

1) DCGI – license for operating in India

2) ISO Certification: International Organisation Standards Certificate.

For Example ISO 9000 (almost all companies have it)

This is important to check:

Either **AABB** (American Association of Blood Banks) or **FDA**: (Food and Drug Administration) certification is a must for the cord blood bank to have.

At least one of the above 2 is a MUST for the safety and standards.

You can find the accreditation standards maintained by a particular blood bank by opening its official website and clicking on "About Us" or something to that effect.

Stem cell banks usually wear these standards like a badge of honor and place them prominently.

e. Type of Technology

Now that we have moved accreditation standards out of the way, it is time to get to the nitty-gritty of the matter.

If you are serious about storing your baby's cord blood, you will probably end up in the middle of presentations being given out by various cord blood banks.

If there is one thing in common between all the banks, then it is their firm belief that their particular processing method is the most advanced and hence, the best in the country!

They will even provide scientific papers which serve to emphasize that firm belief.

Fear not.

Before breaking down the various processing methods, it is VITAL to understand a few technical details.

TNCs

The most critical factor influencing the storage of your baby's cord blood is the **Total Nucleated Cells** (TNCs) count.

The number of TNCs in the cord blood indicates the number of **potential stem cells available for transplant in the future**. Higher the number of TNCs, **the better** the chance of a successful transplant (if and when it is needed).

1 ml of the precious cord blood contains **8.6 million TNCs**!

The volume of cord blood available for collection at the time of birth usually **varies from 20–200 ml**. For storage purposes, cord blood banks prefer collecting at least 26.5 ml to 40 ml of cord blood.

Storage volume is dictated by the fact that patients suffering from say, cancer will need at least **25 million TNCs per kilogram** of his/her body weight.

CHILD

If a patient needing a cord blood transplant weighed 10kgs, then he/she would need at least 250 million TNCs (or roughly **30 ml of cord blood**) for a decent chance to survive.

ADULT

On the other hand, if the patient needing a transplant is an adult (leading to weight more than 30-40kgs), then the stem cell transplant takes place in 2 rounds.

ROUND 1

His/Her cord blood stored at the time of their birth.

ROUND 2

Cord Blood sourced from either a sibling or relative whose cord blood has been stored in a private bank or by getting a donor match at a public bank.

Siblings and relatives tend to have a decent chance of being good stem cell donors.

f. Check for the financial stability of the Cord Blood Bank

Any commercial activity can go bankrupt. Cord blood banks need to survive for decades, before being financially stable. You must check the insurance plan of the blood bank must. You must ask about the insurance coverage in case of business failure or a natural disaster?

Who are the financial backers of the bank? Is it a subsidiary of its parent company?

What kind of hospitals or research institutions is it affiliated with?

Predicting the future is very tough. It's best if the blood bank of your choice manages to survive at least 20 years in an incredibly competitive business environment.

g. What specific questions should I ask about a Cord Blood Bank I'm considering? Understanding the Banks' Terms & Conditions

Once you identify a Bank, here are some questions you need to ask:

✓ Does the Bank meet federal, state, and accreditation requirements?

The FDA now regulates and inspects family cord blood banks nationally. All banks must comply with these federal regulations or be shut down.

Also, AABB certification and DCGI certification is a must for all Indian Cord Blood Banks.

We must also check what other certifications are carried by the Cord Blood Bank and what is the significance and meaning of the same.

Please Note: The process of registering with an accreditation agency and getting inspected can take a year, so it is understandable if a brand new lab does not have an accreditation yet.

✓ Does the Cord Blood Bank provide shipping with thermal integrity?

Shipping the cord blood to the laboratory is the crucial first step in safeguarding your baby's stem cells. Once cord blood is collected, the blood cells and stem cells in it gradually begin to die. Exposing the cord blood to temperature extremes, either too hot or too cold, speeds up cell death.

Firstly, the kit bag in which the stem cells would be transported needs to have a temperature tool to maintain and measure the temperature conditions inside the box. The standard procedure for transporting fresh cord blood is to keep it within an ambient temperature range of 15 °C (59 °F) to 25 °C (77 °F). The collection kit box is usually sent via air cargo or priority shipping services, hence the cord blood bank needs to make sure that the collection kit is not sent through the x-ray machine, under special permissions, to make sure that the collected stem cells are not exposed and spoiled in the transportation process.

✓ Does the cord blood bank process cord blood within 48 hours of collection?

Agencies that oversee cord blood transplants have set a limit of 48 hours on time between birth and processing the cord blood for cryogenic storage. So you'll want to make sure your bank processes cord blood within 48 hours after the birth.

The 48-hour requirement isn't usually difficult to meet unless severe weather disrupts shipping or you're shipping cord blood internationally. Still, it's an important detail to verify.

✓ Check whether the cord blood bank has actual clinical experience?

Ask the banks you're considering, about how many of their customers' cord blood has been used for transplants and other therapies.

Experience releasing cord blood for transplants and participating in experimental therapies is an indication that the company is successful with clinical applications of cord blood. It confirms that the blood is being stored carefully enough for the stem cells to be viable when removed from the freezer.

Be wary of a bank that has lots of cord blood units in storage, but has never used a unit for transplant. It could mean that doctors have rejected their cord blood – a warning flag that the bank's procedures are not careful or thorough enough.

If the bank is new, you can't expect it to have accumulated years of clinical experience. However, it's reassuring if the people operating the company have a proven track record.

✓ Is the cord blood bank financially stable and profitable?

Cord blood banking is a business, and businesses do go bankrupt. Fortunately, if a cord blood bank goes out of business, invariably another company takes over the frozen inventory.

While it is reassuring that you're not likely to lose your child's cord blood, it's not desirable to have it moved from one lab to another – and, worse, to wonder whether it was correctly maintained in the waning days of the failed company.

It can be challenging to assess a company's long-term financial future, but here are a few things to look into:

Ask the bank you're considering if it has an insurance plan or partnerships with other companies to cover inventory in the event of a natural disaster or business failure.

Look at the business experience of the company: How long has it been banking cord blood? Is it a subsidiary of a large stable company? Is it affiliated with a hospital or research institution? Profitability and affiliation don't guarantee that the bank will be around in 20 years, but they do make it more likely that the business is being competently managed.

✓ Are the transportation and storage process, and storage conditions able to maintain the viability of the product?

Stem Cells once extracted, are transported to the laboratory in temperature controlled kit bags via air cargo without any x-ray examination so that the viability of the product is secured. These are then tested in the laboratory for genetic and other disorders along with the maternal blood collected after or before the delivery. Afterward, it is processed for optimal cryogenic storage. This involves separating separation of Red Blood Cells (RBCs) & Plasma from the White Blood Cells (WBCs), which contain all the important stem cells.

After the lab testing and other procedures, the cord blood and cord tissues are stored in cryo-preserve containers filled with liquid nitrogen maintaining a temperature of -196 degrees.

To make sure that the temperature does not fluctuate of fall down, there are special temperature control devices placed in each container. Also, the power supply is backed-up with 2-3 different sources of power supply in case of shut-down or power-cut.

The total amount of cord blood collected may vary case wise, but the stored amount of cord blood has been fixed as 26.5ml as per government norms. These are stored in 3 different parts in 3 different containers as 20 ml +5 ml + 1.5 ml.

✓ What is the procedure to avail stem cells when required for therapy or transplant?

When a patient is diagnosed of a disease that is otherwise untreatable and requires stem cell therapy to be performed, the consulting doctor needs to issue a letter saying that the patient's condition requires the use of stem cell transplantation for treatment. With this letter presented to the Stem Cell Bank, the viability and other tests will be performed at the laboratory of the stem cell bank to make sure that the sample can be used by the patient and is viable to generate results for the same.

After this, the stem cells are differentiated and multiplied as per requirement and shipped to the therapy centre free of cost within a stipulated time of 7 days within India or abroad where ever the treatment is taking place. This shipment and transportation facility is taken care of by the Stem Cell Bank, and is free of cost for the agreement holder.

Once received, the consulting doctor further checks the viability of the stem cells before using them for the transplant.

✓ What is the Guarantee or Insurance on the preserved Stem Cells?

Most Stem Cell Banks offer approx. Up to 20 Lakhs of guarantee each for the viability of the stem cells; loss of preserved stem cells due to natural calamities or failure in the storage process, and; medical assistance for the treatment cost.

The point to be noted here is the type of Insurance that is provided by these Stem Cell Banks. Most of the banks provide only with the in-house insurance claiming that the above guarantee will be taken care of in case of any such requirement, but there is no surety that the same will happen at the time of need.

For Example: If the storage facility gets destroyed in the act of any natural calamity, and the company suddenly goes up to the stage of bankruptcy, then in the case of a transplant neither the preserved stem cells will be made available, nor the insurance amount will be given to cover the cost of arranging matched stem cells from a public bank for the therapy.

✓ What type of records do parents receive after storage? What information will parents receive in the final report about their stored cord blood?

✓ Does your contract state that the storage fee is fixed, or it may increase later?

- ✓ Does your Bank provide dual storage for Cord Blood Banking within India?

- ✓ Does your Cord Blood Bank give an option to provide banking facility in abroad?

- ✓ Does the bank reserve the right, in your contract, to change the storage facilities as per their discretion?

- ✓ Does the Bank operate its storage facility, or it is provided by another laboratory?

- ✓ Is the Bank-affiliated with a hospital or a research institution? Does the Bank have its research centre?

- ✓ Is the company involved in biotechnology research and development?

- ✓ What other medical services does the company perform? Moreover, how far is the company successful in that?

- ✓ Is the private Cord Blood Bank a publically-held or a private-held company?

- ✓ How long has the company been banking cord-blood?

- ✓ Who directs the day-to-day business of the company? Many cord blood banks have famous doctors on their Board of Directors, but they are not involved with the day-to-day operations.

- ✓ What is the lab inventory of cord blood collections, both public and private? This speaks to their staff's experience with storing cord blood.

- ✓ How many cord blood collections has the bank released from their lab for therapy? This speaks to their staff's experience with releasing cord blood.

- ✓ Does the Bank have its transplant or therapy centre?

- ✓ What is the geographic location of the storage facility: is it at risk for hurricanes, earthquakes, or other natural disasters?

✓ What type of back-up systems does the storage facility have in case of a power failure?

✓ What type of security systems does the storage facility have? Does the facility have fire insurance and proper safety and security measures?

✓ Does the storage facility have power back up or generators, and monitoring systems in place that ensure a controlled environment all the time?

✓ Does the bank have a good network, accessibility, and tie-ups with hospitals? This is important to ensure that they will be able to deliver your child's stored cord blood cells soon enough when the need arises.

✓ How long should the cord blood be stored? What is the period of viability of the cord blood once it is stored and preserved?

✓ Does the lab/bank inform parents, before storage, if the collection is too small for a transplant, and give them the option not to save it?

✓ What happens when the cord blood collected from the umbilical cord is not enough or as per the storage norms, is it discarded or used for research or any other purposes? Is the agreement still in place if the Cord blood is not preserved for therapies or transplants in the future, in the above scenario? Is the family still charged for the storage and preservation facility for which they have paid in advance?

✓ Is the enrolment fee charged once per family, or for each birth?

✓ Is the first year of storage included in the processing fee?

✓ Are there any professional discounts? Most banks offer discounts to medical professionals and military personnel. Some banks have discounts for first responders or students. It pays to shop for these deals.

✓ Do parents have the option of a partial or full refund if they decide not to store the cord blood for any reason? For example, if the lab tests show contamination and the cord blood should not be saved, what happens? Full refunds are typically only offered in situations where the bank provided staff to perform the collection service.

✓ What happens to the amount that has already been paid, in case either the Cord Blood Bank or the Agreement holder wishes to discontinue the said terms of agreement for any given reason.

✓ Should the family ever need the cord blood, check that the bank does not charge to release it.

✓ Does the lab process cord blood around the clock, or only on selected shifts?

✓ What tests does the lab perform on maternal blood?

✓ What tests does the lab perform for infectious disease markers?

✓ What tests does the lab perform for contamination?

✓ Does the lab ever reject cord blood collections based on the tests of maternal blood, infectious diseases, or contamination?

✓ Does the lab maintain a "quarantine tank" for the storage of blood that might be able to transmit an infection?

✓ What tests does the lab perform to measure the stem cell count of the processed cord blood and the stem cell viability?

✓ Is the cost of shipping included in the contract?

✓ Does the shipping company offer bed-side pick-up?

✓ What instructional tools are provided for the physician and delivery staff regarding the cord blood collection process?

✓ Will the cord blood company actively contact the labor and delivery staff for you – or are parents responsible for keeping them informed and coordinated?

✓ What collection method do they use: gravity drip or blood draw?

✓ What method of processing or stem cell extraction is followed by the Bank? Is it manual, semi-automated or fully automated (Centrifuge, Sepax or Sepax 2 respectively)

The centrifuge method of processing is a manual method of extracting the stem cells, in which a chemical named HES (Hetastarch) is added to extract the stem cells. After the processing and extraction of the stem cells, this solution is again added for the storage purpose to maintain the viability of the stem cell extracted (because of the extraction method being Centrifuge). The drawback here is that the use of HES Chemical increases the chance of GVHD (Graft vs. Host Disease – a dangerous side-effect of stem cell transplant) to a great level, if these stem cells are used for the transplant. GVHD occurs when new cells fight against the patient's existing cellular system, which can be lethal. Since cord blood cells are more adaptable than other cells, like bone marrow, they have a much smaller chance of graft-versus-host disease. Also, there are high chances of internal bleeding and renal failure because of the above. In case, the stem cells are not processed as expected, these is a way to reverse processing and further extraction of stem cells is made possible.

Sepax 1 and Sepax 2 however, are semi and fully automated processes which are better than the manual process. Sepax 1 ensures 70-80% of stem cells recovery using plasma depletion process but still uses the HES Chemical as it is part manual and part automated.

Sepax 2, however, does not use HES or any other harmful chemical for the extraction process and also ensures about 99% of stem cell extraction during the processing. Also, the purity and viability of the collected stem cells is of higher degree as there are no dead cells. Sepax is the most efficient method for TNCs recovery.

✓ Processing: Must cord blood be processed before storage?

The earliest cord blood transplants were performed with whole cord blood. Thus, it is not necessary to process the cord blood to save patient lives. There has never been a prospective randomized trial to compare transplant patient outcomes with cord blood that had been stored whole versus processed. Most cord blood banks, both public and private, now process the cord blood to remove both the plasma and the red cells, and cryo-preserve the remaining buffy coat holding stem cells. Some banks also save the removed red cells and plasma in companion storage. Some banks save a sample of maternal blood.

The removal of plasma is also called volume reduction. The volume reduction enables more collection units to fit in a freezer and requires less cryogenic nitrogen per unit.

Also, the majority of banks remove red blood cells prior to freezing, primarily because these cells often burst during freezing and release iron from haemoglobin that can be toxic. The alternate to removing the red cells before freezing is to wash any broken cells out of the collection upon thaw. Removing the red cells also removes the donor's blood type (the ABO and Rh types). When cord blood goes from a donor to a patient for a transplant, the donor and patient can be compatible on all the HLA types used for transplant matching and still have incompatible red blood types.

✓ What is HLA Type and how is it used?

The term "HLA" is short for Human Leukocyte Antigens, and these are proteins in the immune system that determine whether a patient will react against a donor transplant. HLA is a parameter through which the compatibility of the donor stem cells is checked along with that of the receiver's, so as to make sure that the stem cells do not have any adverse effect or get rejected by the body after the transplant. Briefly, there are 6 HLA types that are important for stem cell transplants: in a bone marrow transplant the patient and donor must match at all 6 (100% match), whereas a cord blood transplant is just as effective at curing patients with only a 4 out of 6 match (67% match) between donor and patient.

✓ At what stage does the Bank perform HLA Test, before storage or at the time of transplant?

The HLA type of cord blood is always measured by public banks, and then the type is listed on a registry that can be searched by patients seeking a transplant. The private bank typically does not measure the HLA type at the time of banking, because it is an expensive lab test and can always be checked later from a testing segment of the stored cells.

Also, while private banks charge us for a variety of reasons, we need to check whether this HLA Typing is free for the child, child's family, etc or being charged separately.

- ✓ How much cord blood is needed for one transplant? Moreover, how many transplants are possible from the stored cord blood and tissues?

The crucial thing is not the volume of the cord blood collection, but the number of stem cells it contains. Transplant doctors develop recommendations based on the Total Nucleated Cell count, or TNC because it is the easiest measure to reproduce between different labs. For treating cancer, the transplant dose should be at least 25 million TNC per kilogram of patient body weight (1 kilogram equals 2.2 pounds). The average cord blood collection holds 8.6 million TNC per mL. Thus, the optimal transplant dose requires harvesting:**1.3 mL of cord blood for every pound of patient weight, -or-2.9 mL of cord blood for every kg of patient weight**

However, as more transplant centers are adopting the practice of giving adult patients "double cord blood transplants" with two cord blood units, it is less critical for both units to have adequate cell dose.

- ✓ Are related donors better for transplants?

The overall answer is yes, but this is a complex topic. The two important measures of patient outcome are long-term survival and the impact on the quality of life from graft-versus-host disease (GvHD). Sibling donors tend to trigger less GvHD. Also, sibling donors are available faster than searching for an unrelated donor, and patients have better survival when they go to transplant faster after diagnosis.

The exact comparison of outcome between sibling or unrelated donor varies with the patient diagnosis. For many cancers, the outcomes are comparable, although sibling donors have a slight edge. The largest study was by Weisdorf et al. 2002, for over 2900 patients with CML leukemia. When correcting for all other factors, the survival with sibling donor vs unrelated donor was 68% vs. 61%. Sibling donors show a significant improvement for pediatric cord blood transplants of hereditary disorders. The European Blood and Marrow Transplantation Group (EBMT) reported three year survival rates of 95% from a sibling donor vs. 61% from an unrelated donor.

✓ How much blood and stem cells does a typical umbilical cord hold?

The median size of cord blood collections in private banks is 60mL or 2 ounces. That small volume of liquid corresponds to 470 million Total Nucleated Cells (TNC) or 1.8 million cells that test positive for the stem cell marker CD34. Thus, most healthy full-term babies have over a million blood-forming stem cells in their umbilical cord blood. By comparison, most public cord blood banks will only keep collections that are much bigger than average, and throw out the donations that are below a threshold of a billion TNC, corresponding to a blood volume of about 90-100 mL or 3 ounces.

✓ If I banked privately for one child, do I need to do it for additional children?

All the reasons that you banked for the first child are still valid for additional children.

1. If you want the baby to have the option of using his/her cells, then you need to bank them.

2. If you are banking to cover siblings, then the ability to use cord blood from one child for another depends on whether they have matching HLA type. Two full siblings have a 25% chance of being a perfect match, a 50% chance of being a half match, and a 25% chance of not matching at all. For a cord blood transplant, donor and patient must match at 4 out of 6 (67%) HLA types. The more siblings with banked cord blood, the more chance that they cover each other for possible transplants or other therapies for which sibling stem cells are accepted.

✓ What is the cost of storing stem cells at a decent stem cell bank?

The minimum initial processing and storage fees charged by a stem cell bank in India starts with Rs 9,900/- but that is just the beginning. After the initial charges, the banks also charge per year storage fees for the basic plan. There are 'n' number of plans in which different services are provided and a decent plan with the mandatory or important services that are required, would ideally cost somewhere between Rs 50,000/- to Rs 1,00,000/- but the plans go further up to Rs 3,00,000/- also.

Some of the banks charge separately for the dual storage, while others don't. Another element to look into would be the amount of medical assistance, insurance, and guarantee provided by these banks in case of need. Moreover, the guarantee to arrange for an additional amount of cord blood cells as required in case of a transplant for the child or immediate family, and if the bank is charging for the same (which should not be charged typically).

✓ What plan should you choose?

Most banks have started offering a lifetime plan along with their other yearly plan and 21-year plan. Though it seems very much attractive in terms of cost-saving, there is a glitch we need to look upon. In spite of offering the lifetime plan on papers, there is no mention of the same in the contracts, and there is no guarantee that the services and the facilities will be made available for a lifetime.

It is advisable that we do not fall prey to such promises, and go with the 21-year plan that has been approved as per government norms, and extend the same in future, as and when needed.

Apart from this, there is another important aspect we need to note. Most plans offer to store only Mesenchymal Stem Cells (MSCs) which are derived from the umbilical Cord Tissues and do not even mention or inform that the preservation and storage of HSCs and EPSCs will not be covered under the low-budget plans. It is later, at the stage of transplant, that we will realize that the cost was rather high as we did not preserve the necessary for the sake of paying a little lesser.

The amount of MSCs stored also differs as per the plan. Moreover, some of the banks do not store EPSCs at all. We need to probe and find out the best possible plan according to the insurance we would like to have for our family.

h. Make up your mind before finalizing on the bank where you preserve your baby's stem cells

Deciding on a particular stem cell bank is rather a challenge as there are many things that one needs to consider before finalizing the bank where the precious stem cells of your baby will be banked, preserved and taken care for the future.

Once you have finalized on a particular stem cell bank as per your understanding, made payment and all the other necessary arrangements ready for the process to happen when the baby is born, it is usually time to relax as the major part has been finished from your side. However, in case you would wish to change your bank and choose another one, you still have time until the cord blood has been collected, processed, and stored.

Once the cord blood has been processed and sent for preservation, even though possible with some banks, it is not suggested that you change the original place of storage and preservation. This is only because the stored product has been processed and preserved as per one company's clinical methods and standards, and changing the bank would mean reprocessing, transportation, re-examination and other necessary procedures to be followed, which may lead to the contamination of the stem cells and/or loss in the viability due to lack of proper transportation facilities, change in temperature, etc.

Hence, it is advisable that you take all your time in the world, before finally storing and preserving the stem cells of your baby with a particular bank. Changing your mind, later on, may cost you not just monetarily, but also otherwise.

V. Types of Stem Cell Banking

a) **Umbilical Cord Blood:**

The portion of the blood of a fetus that remains in the Amniotic Sac or Umbilical Cord after delivery of the Child. Umbilical Cord Blood is normally rich in multipotent Hematopoietic progenitor cells.

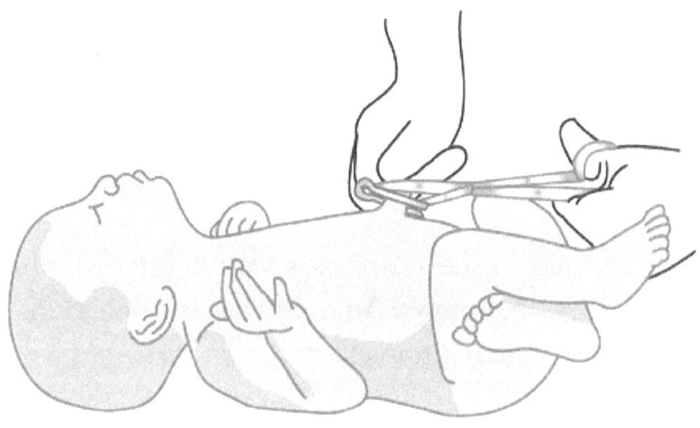

The cord blood is an easily accessible source of stem cells that can be used in a variety of ways.

Umbilical Cord Blood Banking

Umbilical Cord blood: Umbilical cord is the cord connecting the mother and the fetus, through which the baby gets nourishment and all the other important nutrients to grow while it is in the womb of his/her mother. The blood that remains inside the umbilical cord after the baby is born and the umbilical cord is cut is called the umbilical cord blood. The extracted blood from Umbilical Cord and placenta of the baby contains **Hematopoietic stem cells** that help cure genetic as well as blood-related diseases and disorders. Stem cells collected from the available amount of cord blood are preserved without expansion, for future use.

b) **Umbilical Cord:**

A Flexible cordlike structure is connecting a fetus at the abdomen with the placenta, which provides nourishment to the fetus and removes its wastes, during pregnancy. It is a rich source of pluripotent Mesenchymal progenitor cells.

Umbilical Cord Tissues: Umbilical cord also contains tissues that can be stored for future use, as it is rich in Mesenchymal stem cells that are differentiated and expanded for the treatments relating to spinal cord, neurological problems, heart, kidney, liver, etc. and Epithelial Stem Cells that are differentiated and expanded for treatments relating to internal and external skin, diabetes, upper layer organs, cosmetic surgery, etc.

c) **Amniotic Sac:**

A bag of fluid inside a woman's womb (uterus) where the unborn baby develops and grows. Amniotic Sac is a rich source of pluripotent Mesenchymal progenitor cells.

d) **Amniotic Fluid:**

The fluid present inside the Amniotic Sac. It regulates temperature, acts as a shock absorber, and Provides nourishment to the growing fetus. Amniotic fluid is a rich source of pluripotent Mesenchymal progenitor cells.

e) **Dental Pulp:**

The dental pulp is the soft tissue inside a tooth. It is rich in powerful Mesenchymal stem cells of neuroectodermal origin, which have the best chance of giving rise to nervous tissue than any other source.

f) **Adipose Tissue:**

Body tissue containing stored fat. It cushions and insulates vital organs, but an excess of it leads to obesity and other related medical problems. It is rich in pluripotent Mesenchymal progenitor cells.

g) **Bone Marrow**:

A Spongy tissue present in the hollow cavity of the bones. It contains pluripotent mesenchymal progenitor cells.

h) **Menstrual Blood**:

The flow of Blood from the uterus which occurs at monthly intervals during a female's reproductive cycle. It is rich in pluripotent Mersenchymal progenitor cells.

VI. Understand the Contracts

In the above list of questions that were mentioned under the most important points to be considered, we have mentioned the details that one must consider before finally deciding Stem Cell Banking with a particular Bank of choice.

Ideally, the terms and conditions of the agreement are mostly same as the answers to the above questions, but, some of the contracts may differ slightly and state otherwise in writing, and also communicate that all other details mentioned apart from the agreement will not be counted. Hence, it is very important that you read the agreement points very carefully, and also discuss the same in detail with your family as well as the company representative, in case of any missed or non-communication from the Bank's side.

There are certain things we must note on priority:

☐ Some Banks mention in their contract that the collection and initial transportation of the cord blood, cord tissue and the maternal blood will be the responsibility of the Client, and only provide the client with a list of Do's and Don'ts inside the collection kit bag. The physician needs to be paid for the collection and contamination or loss of the product in any form during collection and transportation is not the guarantee of the Bank.

However, in such cases, there is another clause in the agreement stating that if there is **prior information and intimation or request from the client's side**, then the **collection and / or transportation** part will be taken care by the Bank, at no extra cost.

☐ The **Bank reserves the right to shift the preserved stem cells** from one centre to another at their own cost and risk, and in such a case they promise to inform the same to the client within a period of about 14 days.

☐ Banks that have a **dual storage facility** do not offer the storage of stem cells at two locations by default. This facility needs to be availed at an extra cost on demand.

☐ There are different plans that Banks offer along with different storage terms for a particular period, ranging from one year, **21 years**, or lifetime. The agreement and payment details, along with other terms & conditions, must confirm the same in the written agreement.

☐ The medical assistance and insurance are given by the Bank must be checked, whether it is just a guarantee given from the Bank's side, or it is insurance taken and provided from a particular **insurance company** for medical purpose.

☐ In case of any such need, if the agreement needs to be terminated from either the Client's side or the Bank's side, check for the **procedure to do so and the eligibility of the refund amount**; and, what happens to the product after that in such a scenario. Check for the cancellation fees that will be charged.

☐ For Transplant purposes - Some of the Banks suggest in the agreement, that the viability testing would be done and judged as per the set standard of the Bank, which may not prove **viable when tested at physician's end**. What support would be provided by the Bank if the viability of the product becomes questionable in such a case where a transplant is needed? Will the Bank arrange for Stem Cells from a Public Bank on their own cost? Will the Bank pay for the **medical assistance**?

☐ What is the **level of ownership, responsibility, and guarantee** that the Bank offers to take regarding the product in writing, at each level?

☐ At what time will the **HLA Typing and CFU Typing** be performed?

☐ Check for the **after sales assistance** details mentioned in the contract

The Agreement clauses with all the mentioned Terms & Conditions need to read and understood very carefully before signing, to avoid regretting a valuable decision in the future.

We wish you all the best and a disease-free life for you and your family.

Choose Well!

Terminology

Stem-cell therapy is the use of stem cells to treat or prevent a disease or condition. Stem cells are being studied for several reasons. The molecules and exosomes released from stem cells are also being studied to make medications.

With decades of research work, we have found the cure for many incurable diseases, and we are still on our way to explore and find possible new cures for other untreatable diseases.

Research with stem cells

Scientists and researchers are interested in stem cells for several reasons. Although stem cells do not serve any one function, many can serve any function after they are instructed to specialize. Every cell in the body, for example, is derived from first few stem cells formed in the early stages of embryological development. Therefore, stem cells extracted from embryos can be induced to become any desired cell type. This property makes stem cells powerful enough to regenerate damaged tissue under the right conditions.

a. What is a Stem Cell Transplant?

A Stem Cell Transplant is a procedure to infuse healthy cells into the body to replace the damaged or unhealthy blood-forming cells.

Stem Cells acquired from the bloodstream can be used for treatment in two different ways.

There are three kinds of transplants:

1. An **Autologous transplant** (or rescue) is a type of transplant that uses the person's stem cells. These cells are collected in advance and

returned at a later stage. They are used to replace stem cells that have been damaged by high doses of chemotherapy, used to treat the person's underlying disease.

2. In Syngeneic **transplants**, patients receive stem cells from their identical twin.

3. In an Allogeneic transplant, the patient receives bone marrow or peripheral blood stem cells from another person – usually a sibling, but sometimes an unrelated donor.

But it is highly unlikely to find an exact match for the stem cells required by the patient, and at the right time when it is required. Also, there are chances that you might get a reaction after the transplant called graft versus host disease (GVHD). This means that the immune cells from the donated stem cells attack some of your body parts. To avoid reacting, the receiver of the donor cells need to have anti-rejection drugs for the rest of his/her life.

b. Types of Stem Cells:

There are different types of Stem Cells:

1. *Adult Stem Cells*

Adult stem cells, also known as Somatic Stem Cells, are undifferentiated cells, found among differentiated cells in a tissue or organ. Adult stem cells can renew themselves and differentiate to yield some or all of the major specialized cell types of the tissue or organ. These cells can be found throughout the body, and their main function is to multiply by cell division to replenish dying cells and regenerate damaged tissues.

Among other various kinds of Adult Stem Cells present in our body, namely Hematopoietic stem cells, mammary stem cells, intestinal stem cells, mesenchymal stem cells, endothelial stem cells, neural stem cells, olfactory adult stem cells, neural crest stem cells, testicular stem cells; below are the 2 most important types of adult stem cells that are currently stored and preserved by the Stem Cell Banks, for future treatment or therapy of an ailment:

i. **Hematopoietic stem cells (HSCs)**

Hematopoietic stem cells are unique cells that mature into several blood cell types found in our body like Red Blood Cells, White Blood Cells, and platelets. Hematopoietic stem cells are found in the bone marrow and umbilical cord blood. They are also called Blood Stem Cells.

ii. **Mesenchymal stem cells (MSCs)**

Mesenchymal stem cells (MSCs) are **adult stem cells** of stromal origin and can differentiate into a variety of cell types, including bone cells, cartilage cells, muscle cells, and fat cells. These specialized cells each have their characteristic shapes, structures, and functions, and each belongs in a particular tissue. MSCs are multi-potent adult stem cells that are present in multiple tissues, including **umbilical cord**, bone marrow, and fat tissue. MSCs available from the placenta, bone marrow, adipose tissue, lung, blood, umbilical cord, and dental pulp tissues, Wharton's jelly from umbilical cord and teeth

- ☐ Optimized protocols and media systems for expansion and differentiation
- ☐ Well-characterized with robust expansion and differentiation capacity

MSCs are attractive for clinical therapy due to their ability to differentiate, provide trophic support, and modulate the innate immune response.

Stem cell function becomes impaired with age, and this contributes to the progressive deterioration of tissue maintenance and repair. A likely important cause of increasing stem cell dysfunction is an age-dependent accumulation of DNA damage in both stem cells and the cells that comprise the stem cell environment.

iii. **Neural stem cells**

Neural stem cells in the brain give rise to its three major cell types: nerve cells (neurons) and to categories of non-neuronal cells – astrocytes and oligodendrocytes.

Neural stem cells share many properties with hematopoietic stem cells (HSCs). Remarkably, when injected into the blood, neurosphere-derived cells differentiate into various cell types of the immune system.

iv. **Epithelial stem cells (EPSCs)**

Epithelial stem cells are considered the key resource for epidermal and skin regeneration and are proposed as a preferential target for gene therapy. Most epithelial tissues self-renew throughout adult life due to the presence of multi-potent stem cells and unipotent progenitor cells. EPSCs in the lining of the digestive tract occur in deep crypts and give rise to several cell types: absorptive cells, goblet cells, Paneth cells, and enteroendocrine cells.

v. **Skin stem cells**

Skin stem cells occur in the basal layer of the epidermis and at the base of hair follicles. The epidermal stem cells give rise to keratinocytes, which migrate to the surface of the skin and form a protective layer. The follicular stem cells can give rise to both the hair follicle and the epidermis.

2. *Embryonic stem cells (ESCs)*

Embryonic Stem Cells are stem cells derived from the undifferentiated inner mass cells of a human embryo. Embryonic stem cells are pluripotent, meaning they can grow (i.e., differentiate) into all derivatives of the three primary germ layers: ectoderm, endoderm, and mesoderm.

Human embryonic stem cells (hESCs) can be used in research to: Improve our understanding of how the body develops from a fertilized egg; this can also provide insights into how our adult tissues are maintained and repaired in health.

However, Embryonic Stem Cells are not used for therapy or transplant, because the stem cells need to be attained when the embryo is only 4–5 days old and doing so would mean damaging and killing the embryo, which is considered as illegal and hence, it is not in practice. For research purposes, however, the in-vitro fertilization (artificial preparation of embryo in the lab) is used.

Embryonic stem cells can become all cell types of the body because they are pluripotent. **Adult stem cells** are thought to be limited to differentiating into different cell types of their tissue of origin.

c. What is Stem Cell Banking?

Stem Cell Banking is the process of Banking and preserving these valuable life-saving stem cells through specified Stem Cell Banks which follow a traditional method of preservation as per the International storage norms and procedures specified for the above.

References

Some of the important websites, from where the information was read and understood, are listed below:

Authority sources

1) American Academy of Paediatrics. Work Group on Cord Banking. Cord blood banking for potential future transplantation: subject review. Paediatrics. 1999; 104:116–8.

2) Sun J, Allison J, McLaughlin C, Sledge L, Waters-Pick B, Wease S, et al. Differences in quality between privately and publicly banked umbilical cord blood units: a pilot study of autologous cord blood infusion in children with acquired neurologic disorders. Transfusion. 2010;50: 1980–7.

3) National Guidelines for Stem Cell Research. Indian Council of Medical Research & Department of Biotechnology 2017. Available from: http://www.icmr.nic.in/guidelines/Guidelinesfor stem cell research_2017.pdf*. Accessed January 21, 2018.

Website resources

- http://www.superbabyonline.com/stemcellbanking/
- http://parentsguidecordblood.org/en/faqs
- http://www.aabb.org/sa/facilities/celltherapy/Pages/cordbloodfaqs.aspx?gclid=COq79svD5s4CFcwPaAod5IQN7A
- http://parentsguidecordblood.org/en/accreditation
- http://parentsguidecordblood.org/en/faqs
- http://www.jeevan.org/about-the-registry/

- https://www.quora.com/Who-is-better-for-stem-cell-banking-in-india-between-Cryo-save-and-Life-Cell
- http://parentsguidecordblood.org/en
- https://www.quora.com/What-is-the-most-trusted-private-stem-cell-bank-in-India
- http://www.parents.com/pregnancy/my-baby/cord-blood-banking/comparing-cord-blood-banking-companies/
- http://www.mostinside.com/cord-blood-banking/
- http://parentsguidecordblood.org/en/family-banking
- https://www.lifeforcecryobanks.com/pdf/Top%20Ten%20CB.pdf
- http://zeenews.india.com/news/health/health-news/private-cord-blood-banks-are-fooling-the-public-say-doctors_1584902.html
- http://www.aabb.org/sa/facilities/celltherapy/Pages/cordbloodfaqs.aspx?gclid=COq79svD5s4CFcwPaAod5IQN7A
- https://www.topteninsider.com/stem-cell-banking
- http://www.indiacom.com/yellow-pages/stem-cell-banks/
- http://www.biospectrumindia.com/biospecindia/news/158210/umbilical-cord-stem-cell-banking-bandwagon-swells
- http://parentsguidecordblood.org/en/news/caricord-signs-marketing-agreement-ascend-therapeutics
- http://parentsguidecordblood.org/en/news/pacificord-healthbanks-biotech-company
- http://www.eurostemcell.org/faq/what-diseases-and-conditions-can-be-treated-stem-cells
- https://www.cordlife.com/sg/treatable-diseases
- http://parentsguidecordblood.org/en/diseases
- https://www.cirm.ca.gov/patients/power-stem-cells
- http://www.stemcellresearchnews.net/Diseases_Treated.aspx

- http://health.usnews.com/health-news/family-health/diabetes/articles/2009/03/13/stem-cells-10-diseases-they-may--or-may-not--cure

- http://www.explorestemcells.co.uk/majordiseasesstemcells.html

- https://fetus.ucsf.edu/stem-cells

www.ingramcontent.com/pod-product-compliance
Lightning Source LLC
Chambersburg PA
CBHW051124250726

48655CB00007B/2879